Facts about Neu
Brief   Patients

Facts about

Neural Therapy

according to Huneke

(Regulating Therapy)

Brief Summary for Patients

Peter Dosch MD

20th (German) Edition
1st English Edition

Translated by Arthur Lindsay MIL MTG BDÜ ASTI

Karl F. Haug Publishers, Heidelberg

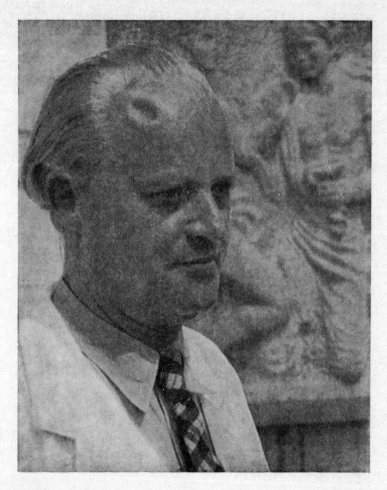

Ferdinand Huneke MD (died 2 June 1966)

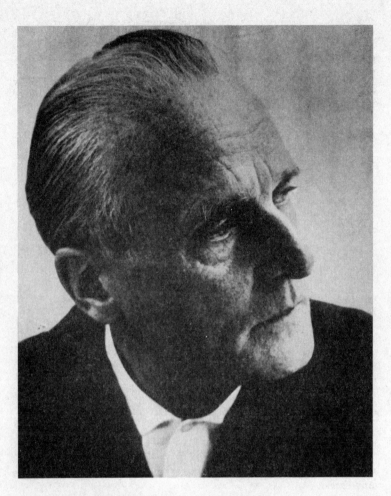

Walter Huneke MD (died 4 March 1974)

Short title:

Dosch, Peter:

Facts about Neural Therapy according to Huneke (Regulating Therapy), Brief Summary for Patients; 1st English (20th German) Edn; tr. Lindsay, Karl F. Haug Publishers, Heidelberg 1985

 ISBN 3-7760-0851-2

Printing history: 1st German edition 1967
         19th German edition 1984
         20th German edition 1984
         1st English edition 1985

Publisher's number: 8573
        ISBN 3-7760-0851-2

Layout by Karl F. Haug Verlag GmbH & Co

Set in 10pt Times New Roman leaded 2pt

Typeset and printed by Pilger-Druckerei GmbH, 6720 Speyer (Federal Republic of Germany)

Preface

> The physician has but a single task:
> to cure; and if he succeeds,
> it matters not a whit
> by what means he has succeeded!
> *Hippocrates (fl. c400 BC)*

I have written this booklet for patients, for they ought to know something about a method of treatment with so great a future. This method is no mysterious form of medical magic, but a living approach to healing that gives those who have eyes to see a reverent but satisfying insight into the secrets of life, it offers new hope to the sick and shows them the way to health. 'Only that is lost which is abandoned!'

Peter Dosch MD
6345 Schwendt nr Kössen (Tyrol, Austria)

Foreword to the 1st English edition

In recent years, man's development of chemistry and of technology has bounded ahead. But this has proved to be a mixed blessing and not always synonymous with progress. Instead, it has begun to threaten his environment and thus his very existence. Too much stress, too many stimuli of every kind, chemical pollution within and without; these have overtaxed and to some extent blocked man's 'vital nerve', the neurovegetative system that acts as the body's life-preserving regulating mechanism and controls the organism's defences and its self-healing powers. Throughout the world, the call grows ever more unmistakable to conserve and live more in tune with nature, and to use more natural, less harmful medical treatment methods with fewer side effects.

In this threatening situation, general practitioners and specialists are increasingly resorting to a low-risk, ecological, and at the same time highly effective holistic method, neural therapy with local anesthetics, discovered in Germany by the brothers Huneke. This method is an efficient adjunct to orthodox medicine, because it can restore dysregulation to normality and cure a wide variety of previously often incurable functional and organic disorders by not merely treating symptoms but by attacking the cause.

On the strength of its far-reaching and sometimes surprising cures, this method has appealed to an ever increasing number of practitioners. And since the publication of the English-language edition of my Manual of Neural Therapy, their ranks have grown worldwide, well beyond the limits of the countries where German is the only or principal language of communication. Because neural therapy depends upon a close collaboration between the informed patient and the treating physician, publication of the English-language edition of this explanatory booklet for patients has become an urgent necessity.

9

For the sick, I hope that this brief summary may point the way to an effective, biologically acceptable method of treatment. If it achieves this, it will at the same time simplify the work of the neural therapist.

Peter Dosch MD

Small causes, great effects

On a bright, sunny summer's day in 1666, the 23-year old English physicist Isaac Newton was lying under an apple tree, dreamily meditating. Suddenly he was jolted out of his daydreams by an apple thudding to the ground beside him. While he was taking a hearty bite, a thought occurred to him: why do all objects fall straight to the ground, as if attracted by some magnetic force? Most of us would not have given the matter another thought, but the young scientist did. And this thought led him to formulate the laws of gravity that made him famous. Physics and astronomy still owe him a great debt for recognizing the importance of this everyday occurrence, by which a genius was stimulated to thoughts that led to a breakthrough which was anything but everyday.

This story inevitably comes to mind when one learns that modern neural therapy owes its discovery to a similar accident, observed and interpreted by a genius. For years, two physicians, Ferdinand and Walter Huneke, had vainly attempted to help their sister who often suffered severe migraine attacks. No matter what they tried for this distressing malady had failed. They might relieve pain for brief periods, but no lasting improvement could be achieved, let alone a cure. On the occasion of a renewed and particularly violent attack, Ferdinand remembered that an older colleague hat recently drawn his attention to a remedy for rheumatism which he had found effective in similarly painful disorders. He quickly transferred the contents of an ampoule of this product to his syringe and carefully injected it into the patient's vein. After their many disappointments, neither expected much from this new experiment. But this time something happened that shook Ferdinand Huneke to such an extent that it simply would not let him go: while he was still administering the injection, the blinding headache

11

simply vanished, together with the flashing sensation in front of the eyes, the dizziness, nausea and depression that are all characteristic migraine symptoms. The patient's pain-racked expression relaxed, and what had only moments earlier been someone full of despair turned at a stroke into a smiling, healthy individual.

Obviously, something totally new had happened; something that was not merely the suppression of pain but a deep-acting cure that had apparently changed the whole person in mind and body. After so many unsuccessful injections in the past, Ferdinand Huneke was fully convinced that this cure could not be the result of suggestion or imagination. He discussed his experience with his brother Walter, and they decided to carry out a number of experiments with the product. As a result, they found that the product used was made in two different forms, one for direct intravenous injection and the other, with a procaine additive, for painless injection into the muscles. Procaine (Novocaine) is a local anesthetic used by dentists, for example, in preparing for dental extractions. For his sister's intravenous injection, Ferdinand had accidentally used the product containing procaine; it was this additive that had produced the startling cure. Until then, it was widely believed that procaine injected intravenously would result in fatal cerebral paralysis. Ferdinand Huneke's mistake had now proved that this was not the case, and that apart from its usefulness as a local anesthetic procaine could also be used as a remedy.

After this discovery, the two brothers continued their experiments with a procaine solution to which they added a little caffeine. This made the product still better tolerated, and further increased its effectiveness. The German pharmaceutical firm Bayer demonstrated the outstanding therapeutic qualities of this compound and launched it on the market under the trade name of 'Impletol'.

12

Three years later, in 1928, the two brothers jointly published a summary of the results of a series of experiments, in which they first carefully tested each injection on themselves to ensure that it was completely free from risk. With the publication of this, under the title of 'Unfamiliar remote effects of local anesthetics', what we now know as neural therapy was born. 'Neural therapy' is the name given to using the nervous system to effect a cure. That the product did not act via the bloodstream was proved by the fact that chronic headache and other painful disorders often vanished just as suddenly when it was injected not intravenously but into nearby tissue. The speed with which the healing processes occurred long before the product could be absorbed was reminiscent of electricity. Only the nerves of the autonomic system could act as the means of transmission, i. e. that part of the nervous system which is not subject to the will. The human organism provides a vast network of the finest electrical circuits for these 'vital nerves', having a total length of twelve times the circumference of the earth. It connects every one of our 40 trillion (40 million million million!) cells with every other to form a living whole. This autonomic (= neurovegetative) system controls the vital processes everywhere in our bodies; it regulates breathing, circulation, body temperature, the activities of the digestive glands, metabolism, hormone formation and distribution; it causes the heart to beat, even when we are asleep, and controls all the numerous automatic processes without which we could not live. We now know that these nerves are the pathways to illness and back to health, and that procaine and other neural-therapeutic products, if correctly applied at the site of a disturbance, are capable of eliminating these autonomic regulatory dysfunctions. By the re-establishment of normal electrical conditions in nerves and tissues, the disturbed functions are also restored to normality, and the patient returns to health as far as this is anatomically still possible.

Illness indicates that the living organism as a whole is somehow out of control. An organ (heart, gallbladder, eye, joint etc) never becomes diseased in isolation, but always the whole individual, in body and soul. The physician's task, not by any means always an easy one, is to intervene here in a regulating manner. At present, mankind's knowledge is doubling every ten years. But this knowledge is still not enough for a complete understanding of the complex cybernetic processes in the living organism. In medicine we still have to rely not upon knowledge alone but also the skill of those who have mastered the art of healing and can draw upon the experience of millennia of empirical medicine, who observe and make effective use of the reactions of the living organism, even when they cannot find complete explanations in modern science of the effects they observe. In medicine above all, success should be the sole criterion: right is whoever and whatever is capable of healing the sick.

Von Hering, a German physiologist, prophesied in 1925 that 'the intelligent use of the neurovegetative system will one day become the most important element of the art of medicine'. The Huneke brothers have shown us an excellent means of making use of it in neural therapy, which is a genuinely holistic therapy. Physicians will have to take a leaf out of their book, if they want to become more successful in helping their patients. Their first commandment should always be: Thou shalt help, to the best of thy ability, thy knowledge, and thy conscience!

Meanwhile, time has worked in favour of the ultimate scientific recognition of the Huneke therapy. At the suggestion of Professor Dr F. Hopfer, an experienced neural therapist, a team was formed in Vienna that set itself the task of carrying out scientific research in medical fringe areas and methods of empirical medicine. This research group included such famous scientists as the professors Harrer, Fleisch-

14

hacker, Kellner and Pischinger. It was able to offer objective proof of the phenomena of neural therapy according to Huneke, some of which had until then been regarded as controversial. According to their conclusions, illness is the result of disturbances in the basic autonomic system, what Pischinger called the cell-environment system. The extremely fine endings of the autonomic nervous system and the blood vessels terminate in the fluid that surrounds every cell. This is where all vital functions, such as metabolism, blood supply, temperature, cell respiration, energy balance, and the acid/base balance are ultimately controlled by the entire nervous system; similarly, when any disturbance occurs in the organism, it is also here that the initial counter-regulatory action can be shown to occur. The Viennese team proved that inflammatory disorders, injuries, bacterial foci, foreign bodies, and scars can produce permanent disturbances in this crucial regulating system; that such interference fields and foci can place the entire human being under strain far beyond their immediate vicinity; and that in such cases the likelihood of the organism's succumbing to illness is increased. Obviously, if there is further damage that can no longer be overcome, illness is likely to occur in organs or feedback control systems weakened by hereditary factors or previous disease. In these studies, differences due to such interference fields were found to occur as between the two sides of the body, in the blood picture, in temperature, in oxygen and energy metabolism, and included changes in the electrical resistance of the skin and in bio-electrical potential. All these returned to normal after elimination of the interference field by procaine and the Huneke phenomenon. These results prove that skilful procaine therapy as taught by the Huneke brothers can completely cure illness by attacking it at its roots.

Segmental treatment: a part of neural therapy

For the first sixteen years of their practice of neural therapy, the Huneke brothers and their many disciples throughout the world used procaine only in the form of therapeutic anesthesia in the area directly affected by the disorder. This so-called segmental treatment was enough by itself to produce some remarkable cures. It can be used to treat a wide variety of symptoms, such as chronic headache, insomnia, neuralgia, rheumatism, sciatica, lumbago, inflammations of the joints; disorders of the middle ear, such as partial deafness; eye disease, eczema, lower abdominal disorders, certain cardiac disorders, asthma, enlarged prostate, gastric disorders; disorders of liver and gallbladder. In segmental treatment, the basic therapeutic processes are related to those used by empirical medicine in the past, in the application of heat and cold, massage, various forms of counter-irritation, and Chinese acupuncture. In this context, procaine has proved to provide a particularly effective and far-reaching therapeutic stimulus.

In a gallbladder colic, for example, the pain radiates from the right costal margin to the right shoulderblade. Hot fomentations on these painful areas relieve the colic pain. Procaine treatment of this area by skin quaddles is even more effective. The practising neural therapist knows that he can therapeutically influence internal organs through certain skin areas; some of these he knows, others he can find. 5000 years ago, the Chinese had already discovered that a patient suffering from a disorder of the liver or gallbladder often has a pressure-sensitive point above the right eye, and they set an acupuncture needle there. Neural therapists have since made use of this knowledge that empirical medicine has transmitted down to us from time immemorial, and have incorporated it in their own method; in doing so they found that if procaine is injected at the correct site, it further increases the

16

effectiveness of inserting the needle. In the Huneke therapy as in acupuncture, the correct site is crucial.

The elimination of pain can produce a chain reaction that leads to a cure. For example, we may have pulled a muscle as a result of a clumsy movement; this causes pain. The pain produces spasm in the surrounding musculature. As a result, the blood can no longer flow as freely as before into the area cramped by pain and muscle spasm. In such an area of reduced blood supply, the oxygen supply is reduced and metabolic waste is no longer removed; both these increase pain. The vicious circle is complete: pain, spasm, poor circulation, more pain, more spasm, and so on. In the end, one-sided muscular tension can cause individual vertebrae to become displaced and press on major nerves, making the disorder more extensive and more complex. This is how a simple lumbago can turn into severe sciatica. But the spiral of pain can produce even more widespread effects: the pain results in insomnia, nervous resistance is steadily reduced, the patient becomes ever more nervous and sensitive to pain. Medicines are prescribed and taken, and affect the stomach; the liver can no longer cope with the demand for detoxification; there is increasing loss of appetite. One thing leads to another, until the entire individual is sick in body and soul. The organism goes ever further down a one-way street and cannot find its way out of it again. The neural therapist can break out of this vicious circle by injections that eliminate pain, and reset the signals to recovery: blood supply is improved, waste is again removed, spasm and stress are relieved, and problems that had seemed insoluble are resolved. This explains why the positive reactions produced by segmental treatment usually continue for much longer than the anesthetic action, and why the effect increases each time the treatment is repeated.

As stated, to be successful, the procaine has to be injected repeatedly to the site deep in the tissues whence the pain originates. Hence, a thorough knowledge of anatomy is essential for this method, coupled with conscientiousness, a certain amount of experience, and mastery of a technique that even the best of physicians first has to learn. The medical profession is still divided between enthusiastic supporters and opponents of Huneke's method. Like anything new and revolutionary, it must first conquer the old. But ever more among those who teach and practise medicine have come to recognize that by using this method they can often achieve better and faster cures than by conventional means. As long ago as 1925 the great French surgeon, Professor Leriche, found that a correctly sited injection of Novocaine (= procaine) was often more effective than major surgery, and called Novocaine 'the surgeon's conservative knife', use of which can often take the place of surgery. Any neural therapist can confirm this daily by his/her successful use of selective, pinpointed procaine injections.

The instant cure by the Huneke phenomen (lightning reaction)

As stated, the therapeutic effect of the local anesthetic in the immediate vicinity of the disorder is valuable in itself; but in 1940, the method discovered by the Huneke brothers was materially expanded by Ferdinand's observation of his first lightning reaction, to which science has now given his name. By his discovery, he opened a new chapter in the history of medicine. The facts on which this is based are capable of shaking to their foundations all earlier views on the origins of many disorders.

A woman with a severely painful inflammation of her right shoulder joint came all the way from Breslau to Dr Huneke's surgery in Düsseldorf. Until then, her condition had resisted all treatment by a succession of first-class physicians. At that time, it was still believed that a (suppurative) 'focus' can disseminate pathogenic organisms and toxic substances via the bloodstream, and that these could cause painful inflammations in one of the joints. For this reason, though in vain, all her septic teeth and her tonsils had been removed, since that is where the focus was suspected to be. As a child she had suffered from osteomyelitis and the bone of her left leg had been opened surgically; this in turn was now suspected to be the focus responsible for her state and it was proposed to amputate the leg.

Dr Huneke gave her an intravenous Impletol injection, set superficial skin quaddles over the diseased joint, and injected his product into the joint and to adjacent nerves. All this had often proved successful in similar cases, but this time it failed and he had to discharge his patient without being able to help her. Fortunately, she returned some weeks later, because the area around the old scar on her shin had become so inflamed that it caused her considerable discomfort. Dr Huneke now merely proposed to give her a few

19

superficial injections to treat only this inflammation on the leg. To his own and his patient's surprise, he now experienced his first lightning reaction: the pain in the shoulder on the other side of her body suddenly vanished, and she could freely move her arm, which had until then been immobilized by pain. This single treatment of the scar on her shin was all that was necessary to effect a permanent cure of her shoulder joint. Needless to say, she no longer needed to have her leg amputated.

This proved that an 'interference field' can trigger a disorder in a remote part of the body, and that this illness could not have been produced by the dissemination of bacterial toxins, for how could they have disappeared in a matter of seconds? A much more likely explanation seemet to be that in this case the scar on the shin had acted as an interference transmitter, sending out the false electric control signals via the nervous system that had ultimately given rise to the disorder. They had produced the inflammation in the shoulder, and kept it active. The procaine injection into the interference field eliminated the interference transmitter and made all the symptoms produced by it vanish completely and at a stroke, just as if the organism's state of disorder had been set in order again by this thrust into the system.

At first sight we cannot quite understand how such an old scar from early childhood should be the cause of a disorder that occurs at an advanced age and at a totally different site. But we are all familiar with the following example from our daily lives: the light bulb flickers, and we replace the bulb; the light still flickers. We call an electrician who chuckles as he tells us that no matter how often we replace the bulb, it will go on flickering because there is a poor contact in the power cable next door. The moment he deals with that, the light shines as brightly as ever. Nor does it matter, whether the defect had been there for hours, a few days, or years. Anyone knows that there cannot be any light on the second floor if the fuse is burned out in the basement. Why should we therefore be so surprised when we are told that a scar on the foot can produce arthritis of the shoulder, migraine or some such? The uninitiated may think that pain and dysfunctions must have their origin where they occur. But our electrical simile can be understood by anyone and is by no means far-fetched. Life is related not only to material aspects but also to energy. The nervous system is a power grid that links all cells and all organs, over which every item of information and all regulating impulses are transmitted and exchanged. Every single cell in the body is a tiny battery with a charge of 40 to 90 millivolts. Any stimulus (such as heat, cold, chemicals, injuries, etc) causes this potential to collapse. The cell's oxygen metabolism supplies it with the energy for immediately recharging itself to the normal voltage. After excessive stimuli (surgery, injuries, inflammatory reactions) it sometimes no longer succeeds in doing so completely. A cell that has become sick due to a permanent irritation has a lower membrane resting potential and can no longer restore itself to normality by its own endeavours. Accordingly, it can not longer fulfil its functions. Such a diseased region, e. g. a scar that has healed but still possesses some residual irritant capability, can send out irritant salvoes that overwhelm the stimulus-absorbing systems and can act as an interference transmitter. Congenitally weak organs, or organs weakened by a previous illness, have a reduced selectivity, like an old radio receiver which receives the signals of several stations at the same time. They process the irrational information from the interference transmitter that they receive together with the correct signals and transform it into pathogenic circulatory dysfunctions and regulatory disorders. Each individual has inherited or acquired weak points, and these are the first to come under stress when an interference field becomes active in the body. This also explains why the same interference field, for example chronically inflamed tonsils, can give rise to totally different disorders in different individuals; one may suffer from articular rheumatism, another may have glaucoma, a third may present with a slipped disk or asthma, and so on. The neural-therapeutic product that the physician injects selectively into an interference field introduces outside energy into tissues whose voltage level is reduced. It recharges the cells and protects them against renewed premature voltage loss. This repolarization by procaine (Professor Fleckenstein) restores the cell's normal functions and switches off the transmitter of interference signals, at least temporarily. When the injection is repeated at the same site, the organism learns to cope better each time with the restoration and maintenance of the correct potential.

Once we are clear in our minds about these relationships, they readily explain why, for example, one-third of all gallbladder patients rapidly have a recurrence of their old symptoms, despite technically perfect surgery; the diagnostic interpretation of this is generally stated to be due to 'adhesions'. However, if the cause of the disorder is not in the gallbladder at all but, for example, in the tonsils, the interference transmitter obviously remains intact after gallbladder surgery and continues undisturbed to send out its pathogenic signals. The gallbladder region can in such a case come to rest only when the cause is eliminated by a procaine injection to the tonsils. But what if there are gallstones present? Almost one woman in two over the age of forty has gallstones, yet only 20 % of them complain of symptoms attributable to the gallbladder. The overwhelming majority live with their gallstones and suffer no pain from them to the end of their lives! In our experience, a high proportion of the remaining 20 % prove to have an interference field that is responsible for their inability to tolerate fats, for colic and other disorders. Obviously, other components also play their part in this clinical picture, such as hormonal changes (pregnancy), and psychic disturbances, such as anger and agitation. The position is analogous for gastric ulcers, lower abdominal disorders, joint disease and many other kinds of illness.

Such interference fields can trigger and maintain in being all kinds of chronic disorders; among the culprits encountered particularly frequently are devitalized, displaced or abscessed teeth; chronically inflamed tonsils; and scars that give no outward sign of anything amiss. But they can occur in any other part of the body, as we shall see later by reference to a number of practical examples. In a Huneke phenomenon, all disorders triggered by the interference field must disappear completely and at once, as far as this is anatomically still possible. In other words, a destroyed joint, rigid as a result of bony ankylosis, can obviously no longer be made mobile, nor can a destroyed eye be made to see again. But the progressive disease process can be stopped, and often it can be reversed to a surprising extent. Obviously, every vestige of pain must also disappear completely.

Unfortunateley, a single treatment is often not enough to eliminate an interference field permanently. We require that a Huneke phenomenon should produce complete freedom from all symptoms for at least eight hours following a 'test injection' to the teeth, and for at least twenty hours when the injection is administered to any other site; repeat treatment at the same site must produce at least the same effect. Experience shows that if these conditions are met, repetition of the same treatment produces ever longer symptom-free periods, until a permanent cure is obtained. This is proved daily by the remarkable cures achieved by large numbers of Huneke disciples all over the world.

We may sum up as follows:

1. Any chronic ailment may be due to an interference field;
2. Any part of the body may become an interference field;

3. Any disorder due to an interference field may be cured by elimination of the interference field, i.e. by the injection into the interference field of procaine or lidocaine (e.g. Xyloneural) or some other neural-therapeutic product.

In what disorders can neural therapy help?

As we have seen, repeated therapeutic local anesthesia (= segmental therapy) can often help, particularly in cases of pain and itching. A faster and more elegant cure can be achieved if a procaine test at a suspect site reveals an interference field and the cause of the disorder can be eliminated by a Huneke phenomenon. We now know that any chronic disorder may be due to an interference field. How often even an experienced neural therapist achieves a surprise cure that he himself had not believed possible in view of the type of disorder, its age and severity. Except for the cases listed in the next chapter, it is always worth trying this novel therapeutic method, especially when everything that orthodox, 'scientific' medicine places at our disposal has been tried and found wanting. The following list is a summary of disorders in which neural therapy has been found particularly successful; it makes no claim to be complete but merely offers a general view of the wide range in which neural therapy has been found capable of making a contribution. Many people have difficulty in accepting that a single product should be capable of offering relief in such a large number of disorders. But in fact what we are looking at is not a remedy at all, but the effect of a product upon the ability of the body to restore itself to health. This is why the injection site is so crucial, for we must activate the organism's innate curative powers and help them effect a cure at the point where the disorder is transmitted and controlled: in the disturbed autonomic nervous system.

Head: Headache, migraine, a sense of pressure in the head; the aftermath of concussion or a fractured skull, such as dizziness, disturbed equilibrium, or post-traumatic epilepsy; cerebral arteriosclerosis; improvement in the patient's mental and physical mobility after a stroke; various forms of circulatory disorders; loss of hair, trigeminal neuralgia, facial paresis, insomnia.

Eyes: Glaucoma; all inflammatory eye disease, such as neuritis, iridocyclitis, keratitis, scleritis, etc.

Ears: Acute and chronic otitis media, vertigo emanating from the ear (Menière's disease), tinnitus, buzzing in the ears, partial deafness.

Nose: Hayfever, atrophic rhinitis, chronic catarrh, loss of the sense of smell, sinusitis.

Throat and neck: Enlargement of the thyroid (goitre) with or without hyperthyroidism (thyrotoxicosis); severe nervousness accompanied by anxiety states, compulsive weeping, etc; chronic tonsillitis, constant sensation of a lump in the throat; whiplash syndrome after motorcar accidents.

Chest: Bronchial or cardiac asthma, angina pectoris, stabbing pain in the cardiac region, cardiac oppression; condition after infarct, cardiac neurosis (nervous cardiac disorders of indeterminate etiology); myocarditis, silicosis, emphysema, certain forms of pulmonary tuberculosis.

Abdomen: Liver and gallbladder disease, disorders after jaundice; gastric and duodenal ulcer, disorders of the pancreas, gastric neurosis, chronic constipation or diarrhea, colitis.

Pelvic region: In women: Inflammation of the womb, fallopian tubes and ovaries; menstrual pain, vaginal discharge; disorders which began after miscarriage

or difficult delivery; infertility, sexual disturbances, morning sickness, tendency to miscarriage.
In men: Enlarged or inflamed prostate, impotence.
Kidney disease; disorders of the bladder, such as bedwetting, irritable bladder, etc.

Joints, vertebral column, muscles: Arthrosis deformans, degenerative disorders accompanied by the formation of bony excrescences; cervical syndrome, spondylosis, osteochondrosis, damaged intervertebral disks; Bechterew's disease, backache, degenerative hip disease (coxarthrosis), lumbago; disorders of the knee, joint and muscular rheumatism, arthritis, coccygodynia; sprained ligaments, torn muscles and their sequelae.
Periostitis (e.g. tennis elbow) after overexertion or accidents, amputation-stump and phantom-limb pain; organic circulatory disorders in arms and legs, post-traumatic osteoporosis, vascular spasm, lymphatic congestion, sport injuries.

Skin: Chronic skin disease (e.g. eczema), painful scars, keloid scars; all types of inflammatory disorders; anal and vaginal itching, hemorrhoids, thrombosis, boils; pain after shingles (herpes zoster), warts, slow-healing wounds; varicose ulcers.

Nerves: All forms of neuralgia, neuritis, sciatica; depression after illness or surgery; 'nervous' organ-related disorders, emotional disturbances, functional disorders; all types of painful conditions.

General disorders: Allergies, neurodystonia, pathological premature ageing; degenerative disorders, sudden loss of performance, post-operative disorders; hormonal dysfunction, weather sensitivity, etc.

What disorders cannot be cured by neural therapy?

The therapeutic range of procaine or lidocaine is very wide, but neural therapy is not a cure-all. Experience to date suggests that the following cannot be cured or substantially improved by the Huneke method:

1. **Mental disease** such as schizophrenia, manic-depressive illness, dementia, and hysteria; these properly belong to the psychiatrist's sphere.

2. **Emotionally induced disorders** in which excessive mental stress (anxiety, worry, fright) have permanently affected the patient's mental balance; these require the help of a psychiatrist or psychotherapist capable of finding and eliminating the psychological interference field.

3. **Deficiency diseases:** When the body lacks one of its building blocks, such as a vitamin or a hormone, this has to be provided from outside.

4. **Hereditary disease,** such as hereditary blindness or deafness, hereditary epilepsy etc; but epilepsy that occurs after head injuries often responds very well to neural therapy.

5. **Advanced infectious diseases,** such as terminal tuberculosis. In these disorders, neural therapy can merely relieve pain and the distressing shortness of breath. On the other hand, unilateral pulmonary tuberculosis has often proved to be due to an interference field.

6. **Complete cicatrization with mature scar formation,** such as Parkinson's disease (shaking palsy after encephalitis), muscle atrophy after infantile paralysis many years previously, advanced nephritis and renal atrophy, and cirrhosis of the liver. Multiple sclerosis responds only rarely to neural-therapeutic treatment, and the same also applies to transverse lesion of the cord (paraplegia), but the patient's

mental and bodily mobility can often be improved by neural therapy in hemiplegia after a stroke (apoplexy and cerebral embolism) if treatment is not unduly delayed; treatment given only years later is useless. At the same time, such treatment is also a useful prophylaxis against the recurrence of strokes. The principle that applies here is that whatever is dead cannot be brought back to life, but damaged cells still capable of regeneration can be saved if the blood supply can be improved.

In doubtful cases, the decision must rest with the physician practising neural therapy who is familiar with some of its technically more difficult injections.

7. **Carcinoma:** Cancer cannot be cured by procaine alone. But we consider that this disease can occur only if there is a predisposition present in the patient and the regulating functions break down because they have become overloaded. If the energy metabolism is inhibited by an interference field, the cell respiration which depends on the metabolism will suffer. In many cases, the cell is where fermentation begins and the cancer forms. The cancer cell becomes disconnected from the autonomic power grid; it escapes from overall control, begins to proliferate in defiance of all biological laws and starts to expand by destroying adjacent cells. The first task must therefore be to reinstate the autonomic control mechanism, to restore normal innervation to the cells, and to make them again capable of receiving their vital supplies of oxygen and other building blocks. Hence, the most important task is first to remove the noxious stimuli that facilitate the development of cancer, particularly those blocking the autonomic system, by eliminating any interference field present. This is the best way to mobilize the organism's self-recuperating powers that had previously been laid low. All other measures (surgery, radiation treatment, dieting,

detoxication, chemotherapy, immunobiological methods, etc) can be effective only if the organism's own defences in the basic autonomic system have first been reactivated. Procaine cannot cure cancer, but there can be no doubt that for us the road to a cure first passes via neural therapy according to Huneke.

8. **Biological effects,** such as those of climate and geopathic influences to which the patient reacts with illness.

9. **Parasitic diseases,** such as worms and their larvae, amebae, lamblia, trichomonal infections; and animal infections communicable to humans, such as psittacosis, toxoplasmosis, etc.

What the doctor needs to know before beginning to treat a patient with procaine or lidocaine

The patient's medical history and the accuracy of what he/she tells the doctor about previous illnesses, injuries (e.g. scars) and surgery can be crucially important for a cure. It is therefore advisable to think about this calmly and to make brief notes. The list should be in chronological order from birth, and the beginning of the present illness should be noted in its proper place. Did this disorder arise after another illness, an accident, an operation etc?

Special attention should be paid to the following:

1. **Tonsils:** Diphtheria, scarlet fever, frequent attacks of tonsillitis, acute abscesses of the tonsils. Have the tonsils been removed by guillotine or enucleation? Do you have enlarged adenoids? Bad breath? The sense of a lump in the throat? Even the specialist cannot tell simply by looking at the outside of the tonsils whether they are acting as an interference field or not.

2. **Teeth:** Next in frequency to the tonsils, diseased teeth are the interference field most often encountered. Not only a tooth with an apical reaction, but any devitalized or displaced tooth can turn into an interference field, even if it is not painful. Has a root abscess been removed surgically (by root resection)? Which tooth is occasionally painful? Are there any septic alveolar pockets? A displaced wisdom tooth? If you have any dental x-rays, bring them with you.

3. **Scars:** Even the smallest scar may be important! When did you have an operation? Have you had an injury? Have you had a lesion that went septic or took a long time to heal, or has an injury given you a lot of pain? Have you had any inflammation or an abscess after an

injection? Is there a scar that occasionally becomes inflamed or itchy? In this context, head scars are particularly important. Scars after bone fractures, boils and carbuncles? Painful corns? Plastic surgery? Look carefully at yourself, you will find scars a-plenty!

4. **Brain:** Cerebral concussion, encephalitis, meningitis; were you a forceps delivery?

5. **Ears:** Have you suffered from runny ears? Do you suffer from a chronic infection of the middle ear? Did you have perforated ear drums; ear surgery? Have you had mumps?

6. **Paranasal sinuses:** Maxillary sinusitis? Has your specialist irrigated your sinuses? Do you suffer from chronic catarrh with a discharge of pus, especially unilaterally? Headaches over one eye? Have you had surgery for a displaced nasal septum? Nasal polyps?

7. **Chest organs:** Have you had pneumonia, wet or dry pleurisy, pulmonary tuberculosis, operations or injuries to the lung, pulmonary embolism? Endo- or myocarditis, cardiac infarct? Thoracic surgery?

8. **Abdominal organs:** Have you had jaundice; inflammation of the gallbladder, gastric ulcer, dysentery, cholera, typhoid, or some other abdominal disorder; an occasionally grumbling appendix? As an infant, did you ever have an attack of diarrhea and vomiting that could have cost you your life, or inflammation of the umbilicus? Food or other poisoning; kidney disease; chronic diarrhea or constipation?

9. **Pelvic region:**
   a: **Women:** Have you had gonorrhea, inflammation of the pelvis, menstrual disturbances, heavy discharge, a miscarriage (with or without fever)? D&C (why?),

how many pregnancies? Forceps delivery, breech births, difficult labour with perineal tears or episiotomy); pelvic surgery (including any from the vagina)?

b: **Men:** Have you had venereal disease? Do you have to get up regularly at night to pass water? Have you any prostate trouble? Have you had any pathological condition of the testicles, epididymis, or foreskin?

10. **Bones:** Have you had any bone or gunshot fracture, painful contusion of the coccyx, periostitis or osteomyelitis? If you have had pleurisy, were any ribs resected? Have you had any bone surgery, a finger or toe joint amputated? Have you had Scheuermann's disease, tennis elbow or something similar?

11. **Thrombosis:** Have you ever had inflamed varicose veins, or ulcers on legs or feet? Where was the seat of the inflammation? After an injection, has á hard knot formed anywhere in deeper tissue?

12. **Foreign bodies:** Shrapnel, broken needles, glass, grains of sand, bone plates etc? Has your dentist used different metal compounds for fillings? Do you have a cardiac pacemaker?

13. **Also important:** In addition, your doctor should also be told about the following:
    a: Are you at present taking any anticoagulants or other products prescribed after thrombosis, embolism, or cardiac infarct? How was your last coagulation-time test? Very low coagulation test values contraindicate deep injections, or your physician may have to give you vitamin K prophylactically; in any event, you must inform your neural therapist if you are taking anticoagulants of any kind.

b: Have you taken or been injected with cortisone or products containing cortisone during the last six months or so? Or taken phenylbutazone or psycho-pharmaceutic preparations, including any frequent or regular use of sleeping pills or tranquillizers? Procaine is compatible with any preparation, but these products have a long-term inhibiting effect on the organism's self-healing powers, which neural therapy has the function of stimulating and unblocking.

c: Have you had any radium insertions or deep x-ray treatment?

The neural therapist plans the treatment in accordance with the information obtained in the patient's clinical history.

A: The physician may decide to use segmental therapy, and treat the patient's disorder by injections into the skin over painful areas; or into deeper tissue where connective tissue has become inflamed, and into indurated zones (fibrositic nodules) and the affected muscles. Or the neural therapist may inject the neural-therapeutic preparation, with its function of normalizing the autonomic nervous system, into or next to blood vessels and nerves; to nerve-exit points, tendon attachments, and periosteum; to and into joints; to peritoneum and pleura, the sympathetic chain (the 'vital nerve') and its ganglia; or to other points based on his/her experience, or adopted from empirical medicine (acupuncture, massage, Head's zones, chiropractice, etc), or those indicated by the patient. For this, the neural therapist needs special training, a good knowledge of anatomy, a special flair and sensitive fingertips, the highly developed sense of responsibility proper to a medical practitioner, and a feeling for the human body as a complete entity, coupled with a technique that has to be learned and used with skill. If every effort in the segment fails, i.e. in the immediate vicinity of the illness, and if this treatment does not produce an improvement to satisfy both doctor and patient, then a search for a possible interference field has to be undertaken.

B: The doctor will test possible interference fields in their order of probability, by selective procaine or lidocaine injections. This is rather like asking them in turn which of them is the active interference field responsible for the disorder in question, that is blocking the body's regulating mechanisms and self-healing powers, and is preventing them from becoming effective. Among other possibilities, the interference field may be one of the following: tonsils; devitalized or diseased teeth; skin, nerve, or bone scars; residual conditions of incompletly resolved inflammation of the liver, gallbladder, stomach, womb and ovaries, prostate, paranasal sinuses, ears etc. If the physician finds the culprit, the result will be the gratifying lightning reaction (Huneke phenomenon). If the symptoms recur, repeat injections may prove necessary in order to achieve a complete and permanent cure, sometimes of severe disorders from which the patient may have suffered for years, even decades, and that may have resisted every other form of medical treatment, including technically perfect surgery.

Every neural-therapeutic injection is a genuine medical examination that tries to determine whether a remote disturbance caused by an interference field or a locally circumscribed segmental regulatory disturbance is involved. Every injection that fails to produce a positive effect on the disorder is also of value, since it tells the physician to continue the search until the causative relationships are found by a process of elimination. As regards the pathological causes, these investigative injections can often tell the neural therapist more than many an x-ray photograph, laboratory

35

test and expensive equipment-based diagnostic procedures; we regard these as useful tools and have no wish to do without them, but consider that ultimately they usually merely show us secondary changes that have come about as a result of the interference-field effect.

Cures by the Huneke phenomenon
(lightning reaction)

A brief summary of a number of case histories taken from a practising neural therapist's records is intended to show how important the patient's history may be to the discovery of an interference field.

Case history 1: Dr H. S., veterinary surgeon, aged 31
When the patient was brought to me, he had been suffering for two years from flaccid paralysis of both legs, and could no longer practise his profession. At a hospital and two well-known university clinics he had been treated with a large number of medical preparations and methods, and ultimately discharged as incurable. His history told of frequent sore throats, 20 shrapnel scars, and provided the information that paralysis had first occurred about a week after he had accidentally pricked his finger with an infected hypodermic needle. Specialist opinion had stated that such an everyday injury could not have caused his paralysis. Consequently, his health insurance had rejected his claim for compensation on account of an injury sustained in the course of his work.

A test injection to the chronically inflamed tonsils produced no reaction. But a few drops of procaine injected into the injured fingertip, in which no macroscopic change was visible, were enough to make the paralysis vanish completely and permanently in front of our eyes, within minutes of the injection. Had he failed to mention this pinprick with the hypodermic, he would without any doubt have remained chained to his wheelchair for life. Dr S. has now been back at work in his profession for fourteen years without relapse. Needless to say, he himself now uses procaine on his animal patients. He has obtained a number of perfect cures by the Huneke phenomenon and thus offers living proof against the objections of our opponents who claim that our cures are based upon suggestion or that we use some kind of hypnotism. But animals do not suffer from imaginary or emotional disorders. Thus he has proved that the healing action in the Huneke phenomenon has nothing to do with the psyche but is due entirely to organic processes. This is a unique and particularly fortunate case, which had been diagnosed as hereditary paroxysmal paralysis and as a hereditary disorder would have been totally unsuitable for treatment by neural therapy. But it was not a hereditary condition but a disorder caused by an interference field which presented as a hereditary illness. This cure shows that this harmless method may be tried successfully even where some rare disease appears to be involved. But this should not be taken to awaken unjustified hopes that no physician can fulfil.

Case history 2: Miss F. K., agricultural worker
Severe abdominal pain for 13 years, diagnosed as neurosis, i. e. 'nervous gastric disorder', because a whole series of hospital investigations and numerous x–rays had failed to show any pathological cause. Continual treatment by various doctors and non-medical practitioners, several stays at sanatoria and health resorts.

Twelve treatments with procaine to the painful region and test injections to all suspect points indicated by the patient's history as possible interference-field sites were unable to eliminate the pain and the sensation of pressure in the region of the stomach. Repeated questioning about previous pelvic disorders produced vehement denials. Finally, merely in order to leave no stone unturned, I gave her an injection into the pelvic region. This promptly produced a most gratifying Huneke phenomenon, and her disorder was as if blown away. After so many years of suffering and disappointment she could hardly grasp the fact of her release. So, something had to be the matter with the pelvis, after all! Only at this point did the woman remember that twenty-five years earlier she had stood for a whole day in cold flood waters, in order to bring in the hay harvest, and that afterward she had had no periods for six months. Once they restarted, they were very painful. This chill in her youth had left behind a chronic state of irritation in the lower abdomen which, twelve years later, triggered off a stubborn 'functional' gastric disorder. Only thirteen painful years later had it proved possible to cure this by eliminating the interference field that was causing it. The woman then made surprisingly rapid weight gains. Since being treated, she has enjoyed excellent health.

Cases 3 to 7 show that disorders having the same name can have totally different causes and therefore have to be treated quite differently.

Case history 3: Mrs E. O., housewife
This patient came for treatment during a severe attack of asthma. In reply to the question, how long she had been ill, she wheezed painfully that the first time had been in childbed, nine years ago. After a couple of procaine treatments of the pelvis, her asthma had disappeared, together with: chronic headache, chronic constipation, painful periods, insomnia, intolerance of uncooked food, hypersensitivity of the eyes to bright light, and high-grade nervousness. All these were due to a pelvic interference field. In her own words, she has become a completely different person. Interference field responsible for this case of asthma: the pelvic region.

Case history 4: Mr R. T., master baker
After returning from prisoner-of-war camp he developed such severe bronchial asthma, with an allergy to rye flour dust, that he was on the point of giving up his trade. After several futile test injections, a little procaine was injected to

a sensitive nerve scar (neuroma) that had resulted from a wartime hand injury. After a single repeat treatment, his asthma has not recurred in twenty years.

Case history 5: Miss R. E., laboratory assistant, aged 26
Since childhood she had suffered from allergic hayfever and eczema; for the last year she also had asthma. Segmental treatment and tests of all suspected interference fields produced negative results. Further detailed questioning made her remember that as a child she had had a fall on a concrete step which had left a depression in the gluteal muscle (buttocks). She had later fallen on this area repeatedly while skiing, resulting in hematomas and a palpable thickening. In changeable weather, she tended to feel 'a bit of rheumatism' in this nodule. Three injections into it made the asthma disappear permanently. Interference field responsible for this case of asthma: an old hematoma.

Case history 6: U. S., infant
At only six months of age this infant girl fell ill with bronchial asthma. Her chest 'bubbled and boiled', the poor child kept coughing and was always short of breath. This distressing state had gone on for a year when she was brought to me. A single injection to tonsils and adenoids was all that was needed to turn her into a healthy child again. What would have been her fate if this interference field could not have been eliminated? In her case, the tonsils were responsible for her asthma.

Case history 7: Mr F. S., master shoemaker from Rostock
Five years earlier he had had surgery to excise a malignancy in the larynx. After this, he developed such severe asthma that he had to give up his business. Treatment by a number of highly reputed specialists remained fruitless. An unsuccessful search was made for secondary growths, especially

in the bronchial passages and lungs. Procaine treatment in the segment (surgical scar, quaddles to chest and back, intravenous injections, and even injections to the sympathetic nerve in the neck) produced no change; his distressing, irritating cough continued day and night. Finally, the dentist who was consulted found that the x-rays showed a cyst in the upper jaw. A Huneke test injection to this site produced a full success that was all but unbelievable for all concerned. The cyst was then removed by oral surgery and the patient, completely cured, reopened his business. The dental cyst had so continually disturbed the basic autonomic system in its regulating function that the interference field had probably enabled the cancer to take root. Its surgical removal had been the second insult that had allowed the regulating mechanism to run out of control in the weakest organ, the lung, and produce the symptoms of severe asthma. In this case, asthma was caused by dental disease.

These histories (3 to 7) all describe cases where asthma was cured. They demonstrate that five times, the same symptoms were produced by five entirely different interference fields, and that therefore the approach to a cure had to be different in each of these five cases. In one case the pelvic region was the culprit, with a condition that had first occurred after giving birth; in another it was an amputation stump; the third was due to a thickening of connective tissue after a hematoma; in the fourth it was the tonsils; and the last was due to dental disease. But it could just as easily have been any other site. To anyone who thinks in biological terms, it will therefore be obvious why, in such situations, any local treatment confined to the diseased organ (in these cases the lungs) is bound to fail. Such treatment cannot cure the root condition, but merely provides a degree of relief. In different circumstances and in patients with different constitutions, the same interference fields would have produced totally different disorders, and we

41

could have found different diagnoses, such as: joint rheumatism, gastric ulcer, migraine, eczema, glaucoma, 'autonomic
dystonia' (neurodystonia), spondylosis, damage to an intervertebral disk, or practically any other organic or functional
disorder.

In other words, some totally asymptomatic and completely
painfree interference field may so disturb or block the autonomic regulating functions and thus the body's self-healing
powers that health is undermined and endangered. If some
additional stress occurs – for someone who is weather-sensi-
tive a change in the weather may suffice – a wide variety of
illnesses and disorders can develop in organs or regulating
systems weakened by heredity or accident. An illness can
manifest itself only in the place and in the form in which the
autonomic nervous system permits, and can be cured only if
the interference field that produces it can be found and eliminated, allowing the previously blocked spontaneous healing
forces to become effective once more.

This is why neural therapy cannot be applied by blueprint
or rote. The physician must enter fully into the patient's
problems and previous medical history by a conscientious
and stringently individual approach, and with the informed
patient's full co-operation in thought and effort, such as no
other method requires. A combination lock can be opened
only if one sets the right combination. In exactly the same
way, the secrets of the patient's illness and of its causes can
generally be discovered only if the physician, working
together with the patient, can find and eliminate the true site
or sites of the disturbance.

In 1963, Professor Hellmeyer, in addressing the German
Congress of Internal Medicine, made this shattering statement: 'Modern medicine has now put us into the happy position of being able to diagnose about one half of all disorders
and successfully treating about half of these'. Good neural
therapists are generally physicians by vocation and are less

42

than happy to find that the organ-based methods taught by conventional medicine allow them to cure only 25% of all disorders. This is why they have committed themselves to a method that considers it more important to discover what is causing an illness and to cure it; this seems preferable to concentrating merely on providing objective evidence of its effects and giving it a mellifluous Latin name, an approach that is all too often the end of all wisdom as taught at medical schools.

A major German illustrated periodical published the story of what one man's sufferings had been, as related at the 1970 Congress of the Medical Society for Neural Therapy according to Huneke. This patient had suffered from a very painful trigeminal (facial) neuralgia, and submitted to surgery on a number of occasions, but without success. In the end, a neural therapist gave him the long-sought relief with a few procaine injections into the interference field at the root of it, a scar resulting from an earlier stomach operation. This article produced a flood of letters to the periodical's editor from sufferers of the same stubborn disorder, and he sent them the addresses of neural therapists. Statistics collected from 25 doctors who used neural therapy with procaine to treat 639 of these cases (among them there were 121 who had previously undergone unsuccessful surgery) produced the following results:

34% cures
37% substantial improvements
14% improvements
and only 15% failures.

In 267 cases, i.e. 42%, an interference field was found to have caused the disorder or to be materially co-involved as a contributory factor. In many of those who had undergone unsuccessful surgery, a complete cure was no longer possible even after the interference field had been eliminated. The results were therefore less good in this group than among those who had not submitted to surgery. This reinforces our demand that before any major surgery, what Leriche called the 'surgeon's bloodless knife' should first be tried, namely skilled neural-therapeutic treatment.

Case history 8: Mr W. U., employee
For years, the patient had suffered from gallbladder colic, and had made the rounds of all the doctors. He also discontinued neural therapy, because it yielded no immediate results, and accepted specialist advice to undergo surgery. Removal of gallbladder and inflammatory adhesions; shortly after the operation, new colic attacks. He returned and begged for further treatment. In the course of further test injections, I injected procaine into a lentil-sized scar on the shin that had remained after an ulcer that healed: Huneke phenomenon. No further liver or gallbladder disorders in eighteen years. He can eat heavy food, needs no further medication, is fully fit for work.

Case history 9: Mrs E. W., innkeeper
For 12 years, this patient suffered from primary chronic polyarthritis; despite hospital treatment, visits to health resorts, injections, embrocations, radiation treatment, and massage, the disease continued to progress. Previous history of diphtheria in childhood; septic tonsils, followed by tonsillectomy. After an injection into the tonsillar scars and one repeat treatment, this patient has remained painfree for the past twenty years and feels well as never before. All previously stiff joints have become fully mobile again.

Case history 10: Mrs L. K., housewife
This patient had for years suffered from arthrosis of the knee, then there was a sudden flare-up. The knee became

44

swollen and within hours was so painful that she could no longer climb the stairs to go to bed. Occasionally one of her teeth ached to which a somewhat shaky denture was attached. An injection to this overtaxed but otherwise healthy tooth immediately made the knee painfree, and she could again climb stairs. Two days later, without further treatment or special care, the knee had become completely normal again. Over the next three years, the tooth was treated again on four occasions, whenever the knee symptoms recurred, but the tooth could be left in position to support the dental plate.

All this may sound somewhat far-fetched, but I could tell of hundreds of such cases and can guarantee every one. Dr M. in Rotterdam injected procaine into a scar from middle-ear surgery years earlier, in a man suffering from inflammation of the interior of the eye (iridocyclitis), who was expected to become totally blind. A few hours later, the patient had recovered full vision and was in due course released from a training school for the blind.

Four weeks later he started work again as a chauffeur. Some years earlier, the Dutch physician had himself been freed from a chronic weeping eczema covering the whole of his lower abdomen that had for many years made life hell for him; Dr Huneke had treated him by injecting his tonsillectomy scars.

From Los Angeles Dr K. reported that he treated an almost deaf woman for a gallbladder disorder by injecting procaine in the abdomen. After treatment, the pain had disappeared, but she noticed with surprise that suddenly her doctor was shouting at her. Her hearing had become normal again, and for the first time in many years she could hear the ticking of her watch.

Dr S. in K. injected procaine into the tonsils of a 70-year old invalid woman who had been suffering for 45 years, since she was 25, from progressive chronic polyarthritis. In her

45

long life she had vainly tried every kind of treatment. He injected procaine into her tonsils, and she instantly became free from pain. Four weeks, later he repeated the treatment. Now, several years later, this woman is still painfree, and there can no longer be any suggestion of her being an invalid. She is again doing all her household chores and as far as her age allows she still helps with work on the farm.

Despite the fact that some of these case histories may sound like miracle stories, they are real enough. Any physician practising neural therapy can tell of similar cures that sound just as improbable. The history of mankind demonstrates time and again that something regarded as a miracle yesterday can become scientific fact today, and that today's wisdom is to-morrow's fallacy.

What should be noted after treatment?

Immediately after neural-therapeutic treatment, the patient sometimes feels tipsy or dizzy. This may continue for several minutes, and may be more or less pronounced. It is totally harmless and disappears by itself within a short time. But to be on the safe side, patients should stay in the waiting room for half an hour and, before driving home, take a short walk to check on their fitness to drive. Procaine is quickly metabolized (about 30 minutes); lidocaine (e. g. Xyloneural) takes longer. Unless the doctor prescribes it, the patient need not go to bed after treatment. Impletol* contains caffeine, just like normal coffee. Anyone who has palpitations or sleeps badly after drinking coffee may have the same after-effects after Impletol* treatment. This is perfectly harmless and may be overcome by taking a mild sedative.

Normally, the patient feels no after-pains. But if the injection has been given under the periosteum, pain may be exacerbated for a time. The patient can easily deal with this by taking an analgesic. Once this reaction subsides, he/she will normally feel a noticeable improvement compared with the state before treatment or may be completely cured. Occasionally, a patient reports that the pain has shifted elsewhere after treatment. But this is an illusion; the 'new' pain was there before but the more severe pain hid the weaker, which could make itself felt only once the stronger pain had been eliminated.

After injection to the tonsils, the patient may for a day or two have slight difficulty in swallowing, rather like that which accompanies the start of a sore throat. No treatment is necessary.

After injection into the prostate gland (in men), there may be some bleeding from the urethra, and there may also be

---

* 1% or 2% pure procaine HCl without vasoconstrictor

some bloody discoloration of the ejaculate. These are quite harmless, should not cause any alarm, and will disappear by themselves. Any slight bloodletting of chronically congested blood vessels never does any harm. The same also applies to any hematoma that may form after treatment; an injection of the patient's own blood can only help by producing an additional healing effect. On the extremely rare occasions that a patient has a procaine allergy, the treatment may produce an itchy skin rash. The patient should tell his/her physician about this before the next treatment session, and the neural therapist can then use a different local anesthetic, such as Xylocaine, Scandicaine etc that will not produce an allergic reaction and offers similar prospects of success. On extremely rare occasions, unforeseeable complications may occur; in all such cases, the patient should consult the treating physician by telephone.

Occasionally, procaine treatment may act as a provocation to the entire autonomic nervous system. In such cases, a new pain may occur in parts of the body that have not been treated in any way, or pain that was already present may become exacerbated a day or two after treatment. Old interference fields often announce their presence in this way after having stayed quiet until then. For the treating physician, this type of reaction may be a crucial pointer to further treatment. The patient should therefore carefully observe such reactions and make certain of informing his/her doctor before the next treatment session. The following practical example should amply illustrate this:

Case history 11: Mr J. K. master tailor
For ten years, this patient had made the rounds of doctors, complaining of sudden severe pain in the right upper abdomen. He reported that this pain – and this is the unusual part that will surprise any doctor – 'radiates all the way to my face and produces the intolerable feeling that someone is

pulling my upper gums upward, pushing the teeth apart and pressing them forward'. These details fitted no known clinical picture. No-one believed him and he was thought to have imagined his symptoms. The abdominal disorder had appeared about a year after gallbladder surgery and was diagnosed as 'post-cholecystectomy syndrome and liver disease', his jaw condition was labelled an 'atypical trigeminal neuralgia', but this was not the slightest use to him.

When he told me that his abdominal disorder hat suddenly disappeared for three months after a tonsillectomy, I injected procaine into the tonsillectomy scars. This made his abdominal pain disappear by a Huneke phenomenon and, as required, he was painfree for twenty-four hours before his pain returned and was, as he reported, even more severe. Occasionally a patient tells us that an old pain is felt to be stronger than before, once the neural-therapeutic effect (which always continues for appreciably longer that the purely local-anesthetic action) wears off. This does not prevent the neural therapist from repeating the test injection to the same site. Two days later, the scar from the patient's gallbladder surgery, which had not been injected, became inflamed and bright red; a blister formed in one part of it and this now burst. In addition, three shrapnel scars on his left thigh became very itchy. Clearly, the test injection to the tonsillectomy scar had acted as a provocation and produced a reaction in other scars, too.

In the second treatment session, in addition to injecting the tonsillectomy scars, I also injected the cholecystectomy scar and the three shrapnel scars on the thigh. These injections produced another surprise: the abdomen immediately became painfree again, but the three pieces of shrapnel that were still embedded became palpable and began to ache. Whenever the patient touched this area, the ominous pain in his jaw returned spontaneously. If, as I was removing the shell splinters under a local anesthetic, I allowed the forceps to touch the middle one, no matter how slightly, such severe cramp was produced in the patient's teeth that he screamed with pain and begged me so stop. But by this time I had already seized the offending disturber of the peace and removed it before the patient knew what was going on. Then he suddenly took his hands from his face and said 'and now it's all gone, all of a sudden'. The ten years of misery he had suffered, and the reason he had been regarded as neurotic or incurable, were simply as though blown away, as if they had never existed.

Thus, practically any illness may be caused by an interference field, and any part of the body may become an interference field that can cause practically any disorder. In this particular case, a shell splinter had kept quiet for fifteen years before suddenly becoming an active interference field ten years earlier. In this case, there were in fact two interference fields active at the same time: the tonsillectomy scars reacted on the abdominal organs of gallbladder and liver; and only one of many pieces of shrapnel produced a disturbance radiating all the way to the upper jaw, where it produced a disorder that defied credence because x-rays, blood tests, and other investigations showed no abnormality, and the symptoms could not be classified in any known clinical picture. In neural therapy, the patient cannot simply leave everything to the physician but must actively collaborate with him or her. The more intelligent the patient is, and the better he/she can enter into the thought processes of this holistic therapy, observe him/herself, and think along similar lines as the neural therapist, the greater are the prospects of being helped by neural therapy.

When used correctly, neural therapy is completely without risk to the patient. It is compatible with every other form of treatment and medication in progress. For seventy-five years, far greater doses of procaine (Novocaine) have been used in surgery without anyone uttering any sign of concern. Procaine is a local anesthetic that has proved its value ever since 1905; it is not addictive, does not produce eczema or other skin disease, and has no other negative side-effects. Even if it does no good, neural therapy properly handled cannot do harm.

Neural therapists worldwide can become members of the International Medical Association for Neural Therapy according to Huneke, a society registered in W Germany and affiliated to the Zentralverband der Ärzte für Naturheilverfahren (Central Federation of Physicians using Natural Therapeutic Methods), proof that this umbrella organization has accepted the Huneke method as a form of biological treatment.

It is appropriate at this point to repeat that this remedy is effective only of it is administered at the correct site. Applied elsewhere it is useless, though it does no harm, and the local anesthetic effect quickly wears off. But used correctly, the therapeutic action continues long beyond the anesthetic. After a promising segmental treatment (i.e. with injections given in the vicinity of the affected area) there should be a substantial improvement in the patient's condition. When the disorder recurs, the treatment should be repeated. The therapeutic action must increase in duration and effectiveness with each repeat treatment, i.e. the disorder should recur less and less frequently, and less severely, until it finally disappears completely.

If, when suspect areas are being tested, the patient suddenly experiences complete freedom from symptoms, a Huneke phenomenon may have been achieved. Before further treatment, the patient should give the physician clear, complete details whether the disorder disappeared completely immediately after the previous treatment, whether there was merely some relief or whether the treatment remained totally ineffective. If complete freedom from pain or partial relief has been achieved, the neural therapist will also want to know how long (hours, days) this effect continued, since further treatment will depend on this information. False or imprecise information can jeopardize the ultimate therapeutic success. If there is a recurrence of the disorder, it is in the patient's interest to have the injection repeated as soon as possible; one or more repeat treatments should lead to a complete cure (as far as this is anatomically still possible). An accurate and detailed medical history, good observation, and the patient's intelligent co-operation can greatly help the physician, and thus the patient. If pain keeps recurring at a particular site, it is best to mark the place with a tiny piece of adhesive tape.

Patience and trust are also important prerequisites to success. Occasionally a bull's eye may be scored first time, but generally the goal is reached only after longer periods of effort. And sometimes sucess remains elusive. But the patient should never give up of his or her own accord, but wait until either the treatment has been brought to its successful end or the physician advises stopping it. Procaine is no cure-all. The patient needs to be resolute and have no fear of a series of injections; in the doctor it calls for a thorough knowledge of this approach to the art of healing. The patient quickly loses his/her natural aversion to injections on discovering that a few unpleasant minutes of treatment are a small price to pay for a marked improvement or a complete cure. Further, long-term medication is never totally free from risk, and the patient can generally reduce or completely discontinue current medication. But the treatment on which neural therapy is based can help the patient only if it is given at the site that happens to be right for him or her. The correct site must be found by test injections that are as individual as every person is different, often by a progressive process of search and elimination. In different individuals with apparently identical symptoms it may be in totally different places. There are no two identical individuals in this world, nor can there be two identical disorders.

> 'Medicine is not a science but an art, and the true physician is nothing more than a skilful artist.' Lahmann

Rejuvenation through procaine?

Ageing is the fate of mankind. But premature ageing, the sudden loss of vitality and the appearance of tiresome disorders due to age and degeneration must be regarded as an illness.

The tissues change with age, they lose water and dry out. Waste products are deposited, cells and blood vessels calcify and sclerose. The more they do so, the worse becomes the blood circulation and therefore the supply of oxygen and other vitally necessary materials. This reduces the efficiency of cells and organs. As a result, ever more deficiency symptoms appear: the skin becomes wrinkled, eyesight deteriorates; hearing, the memory, and the ability to concentrate all become worse. The heart no longer functions as well as it did, joints stiffen, walking becomes more of an effort; sleep and appetite are reduced. The peevish old man sits by the warm stove and wishes for an end to it all, of himself and of all his disorders. And how enviable, by contrast, is the sprightly old gentleman who has kept his vitality, for whom even old age is still worth living. Why, on the one hand, a blessed old age and, on the other, such a miserable existence beset by premature decay?

Science has shown by animal experiments that the constant intake of minute quantities of nerve toxins, and continual nervous irritation from outside, can lead to the same forms of tissue changes and sclerosis with which we are familiar from the process of ageing. Modern life inundates us with nerve toxins and irritants of all kinds: atomic radiation and x-rays; noise; air polluted by exhaust gases from motor vehicles and emissions from industry; polluted water; foodstuffs full of chemicals; tobacco and alcohol; and a struggle for survival like that of wild animals; with war and the miseries that follow in the wake of war; fear, anxiety and restless activity. If in addition to all these there are interference fields in the body to help upset the finely balanced autonomic nervous system, the tolerable limit can easily be exceeded. The body's self-healing powers can then no longer prevent an illness from establishing itself or stop the premature ageing process. Hence, the autonomic nervous system plays as much a part in the ageing process as in any other illness. What could therefore be more natural than to try and use a type of treatment for ageing that will relax the constantly over-irritated nervous system, restore the inner equilibrium, and so arrest or even reverse these abnormal changes due to ageing?

In neural therapy we possess such a treatment. In his long career Walter Huneke was the first to notice that, after he had treated them with procaine-based Impletol*, older people often stated spontaneously that they suddenly felt twenty years younger. In the course of treatment, their posture, bearing and appearance improved considerably. The same was also true of their eyesight and hearing, and of their bodily and mental efficiency. They became visibly more mobile in every respect and often felt fresh and youthful again after a few treatment sessions. In 1952 he published these observations in his book on Impletol therapy (Impletoltherapie). In this he wrote that in a large number of cases 'proper Impletol treatment, repeated every few months, clearly had a rejuvenating effect on the patient and improved life expectancy'.

This indication is of enormous importance to the whole of mankind, but it received scant notice at the time. Perhaps his book contained too much other material that surprised its readers. His statement was recalled only much later, when the successful rejuvenation work done with procaine by the Rumanian school under Professor Aslan was published and produced a worldwide sensation. This has brilliantly

---

* 1% or 2% pure procaine HCl without vasoconstrictor

confirmed the observations made by the Huneke brothers and made them known throughout the world. Perhaps it was inevitable that this rejuvenating effect produced with a German pharmaceutical preparation first had to be confirmed abroad before German science was prepared to accept it. Professor Aslan ascribed the rejuvenating effect to a vitamin-like substance H3, which she believed she found in procaine. She recommended regular intramuscular injections of substantial quantities of procaine into the buttocks, or flooding the body continually by constant medication with products containing procaine, in order to achieve a generalized effect. But neural therapists cannot agree with her theory and recommended treatment. Based on over 50 years experience of the method developed by the Huneke brothers we are convinced that the injection site is crucial to successful treatment and that no new vitamin is at the root of this effect, but the well-known therapeutic regulating stimulus to the autonomic nervous system to which we apply it. We know that with correctly sited injections into interference fields, into the blood supply and under the scalp, and at other reaction points, we can obtain far more by considerably fewer treatments and with much smaller quantities of procaine than the Rumanian school.

It is worthwhile trying to fight pathological premature ageing and the disorders of old age only if a skilful procaine therapy is undertaken to eliminate interference factors and revitalize the system. The medical prescription of additional vitamins, carefully dosed hormone preparations, or fresh-cell therapy does not absolve any patient from the obligation to live naturally and sensibly in every respect, without at the same time being over-anxious to avoid all of life's little pleasures. Growing old is not diametrically opposed to being glad to be alive.

Legal principles and the physician's duty to inform

Translator's note:
This chapter describes the position in W Germany.
The law in other countries is bound to be different in
detail but probably corresponds in general terms to
these provisions.

Certain newspapers have published sensational articles on
the physician's duty to inform the patient. As a result,
patients are more confused than before. This is the reason for
a brief discussion here of the legal principles involved.

The patient has a free choice of physician and method of
treatment. In the Federal Republic of Germany the law
allows the physician 'freedom of method' and does not stipu-
late that only orthodox methods of treatment must be used:
'The rules of medical science generally or preponderantly
recognized are not accorded any preferential status relative
to the methods of treatment used by fringe medicine not recognized by orthodox medicine or those used by medically
unqualified health practitioners.' In other words, orthodox
medicine as taught at university medical schools cannot
claim that it alone represents correct medical practice. In the
case of neural therapy, segmental therapy has received scientific recognition and acceptance. The Huneke phenomenon,
on the other hand, still remains to some extent controversial,
despite the fact that scientific proof of its occurrence and
effects has been provided by several methods.

However, the physician may not use his/her method in an
unlimited manner, but must observe the principles that are
generally recognized by the conscientious representatives of
the method used. If conventional forms of treatment are substantially better and more successful than the method used,
the physician must not persist with his/her method. The
pros and cons of the competing methods must be weighed
objectively in the patient's interest, but to a conscientious

physician this should in any event be a normal principle constantly applied.

Before any injection, the patient's consent is necessary (the legal guardian's in the case of minors). The physician must acquaint the patient of any potential risk that may arise from an injection, but there is some risk in all medical treatment. If general experience indicates that the risk of failure or of undesirable side effects is very slight, the doctor is not required to draw attention to it. A physician's duty to inform the patient extends only to explaining any inherent risk 'in general terms', but a patient may also explicitly waive this right. It is part of the patient's right of self-determination to give the physician of his/her choice a free hand and he/she can choose to be spared the knowledge of all possible complications, if he/she feels that it might merely disquiet him/her. The patient must inform the treating physician in unambiguous terms if he/she requires to receive detailed information beyond the scope of explanations 'in general terms'.

When neural therapy is used correctly, complications, accidents and emergencies are extremely rare. Mutual trust should always form the basis of the relationship between doctor and patient, and this should not be impaired by excessive anxiety or mistrust.